BREASTFEEDING AND MENTAL HEALTH: THE ART OF NURTURING THE BOND THROUGH LACTATION MANAGEMENT.

By

MARY L. ADAMS

INTRODUCTION

Breastfeeding and psychological wellness are pivotal pieces of a mother's prosperity and relationship with her youngster. The administration of breastfeeding, from the study of bosom taking care of to everyday reassurance, is basic in laying out this extraordinary connection between a mother and her newborn child. In the current healthcare crisis, we are learning more about how nursing affects a mother's mental and emotional state.

Breastfeeding gives something other than sustenance. It gives significant profound food to both the infant and the mother. Breastfeeding has been displayed in various examinations to work on a mother's emotional well-being. During nursing, actual association and the creation of oxytocin, otherwise called the "adoration chemical," help ease pressure and fortify the connection among mother and youngster.

Be that as it may, nursing isn't basic all of the time. Many moms endure hardships, for example, locking issues, lacking milk supply, sore areola, or agonizing nursing encounters. These challenges can cause dissatisfaction, uneasiness, and even wretchedness. This is when lactation the board becomes an integral factor. It involves educating and helping ladies in beating these impediments with the goal that they can effectively nurture.

Generally, we're going to dive into how and how we oversee breastfeeding could help the two mothers' and babies' emotional wellness. We look to uncover ways of developing the connection among moms and their kids while additionally supporting moms' psychological well-being by examining the intricate communication among nursing and close to home prosperity.

CHAPTER 1

BREASTFEEDING AND MENTAL HEALTH

Breastfeeding and mental health refers to the association between postpartum breastfeeding and moms' and children's mental health. Breastfeeding has been demonstrated in studies to improve mother and child mental health, although discrepancies call the association or causality between breastfeeding and maternal mental health into question.

According to research, possible benefits include improved maternal mood and stress levels, a lower risk of postnatal depression, improved child social-emotional development, and stronger mother-infant attachment.

Given the benefits of breastfeeding, the World Health Organisation (WHO), the European Commission for Public Health (ECPH), and the American Academy of Paediatrics (AAP) all suggest exclusive nursing for the first six months of a child's life.

Despite these recommendations, it is estimated that 70% of American moms nurse their children after birth, and 13.5% of infants are exclusively breastfed. Breastfeeding promotion and support for moms facing difficulty or early discontinuation of breastfeeding are seen as health goals.

Scientists are still unsure about the specific nature of the association between breastfeeding and certain aspects of mental health. Because research differs in how breastfeeding and its benefits are measured, causality is questionable. Numerous psychological, social, and physiological elements interact in intricate ways that are not fully understood.

Several studies have shown that breastfeeding benefits mothers' mental and emotional health by improving mood and stress levels.

Other studies, however, have shown that the stress of nursing can be detrimental to women's mental health, particularly when pressured with an all-or-nothing 'breast milk is better' mentality. shows a potential impact.

This practice increases mental peace and decreases feelings of anxiety, bad emotions, and tension.
The baby's physiological reaction to breastfeeding reflects this, since it improves maternal cardiac vagal tone regulation, decreasing blood pressure and heart rate.

In conclusion,Breastfeeding's stress-relieving effects are given by the hormones oxytocin and prolactin.
Breastfeeding mothers sleep longer, better, and with fewer interruptions. This practice

has a favorable impact on how the mother reacts to social settings and encourages better relationships and interactions.

Breastfeeding mothers respond to positive facial emotions (such as happiness) more than negative facial expressions (such as rage). Breastfeeding also gives the mother confidence and empowerment because she knows breastfeeding is good for her child.

THE IMPORTANCE OF BREASTFEEDING.

Breastfeeding is beneficial to both the baby and the mother's health. It is also beneficial to your family and society.Nobody else can give your baby what you can. Breast milk is the only nourishment and drink your infant requires. Breastmilk fluctuates with each feeding to meet your baby's needs and stage of development. Breastfed babies are also less likely to become ill than formula-fed babies.

This fact sheet discusses why breast milk is crucial for giving your kid a healthy start in life.

•It is your baby's only source of nutrition for the first 6 months.

•Breast milk is always fresh, clean, and at the appropriate temperature.

•Your breastmilk will alter over time to meet the changing needs of your kid.

•Breast milk protects your kid from certain infections.

•Your baby can feel, smell, and see you when you hold him or her close when breastfeeding.
•This assists you in developing a close, loving attachment with your infant.

Breastfeeding might take some getting accustomed to. It might even be difficult at first. However, the value to you and your child is worth it. Breastfeeding can be started and maintained with the assistance of family and friends.

Babies who are not breastfed are more likely to develop:
•bladder or kidney infections
•stomach and bowel disease (including diarrhea)
•chest infections
•ear infections
•allergies (including eczema and asthma)

•SIDS (sudden infant death syndrome-cot death); •some childhood malignancies; and

•obesity, diabetes, and heart disease later in life.

Breastfed newborns require fewer hospitalisations for infections.

All mammals, including humans, are biologically programmed to breastfeed. Breastfeeding is crucial to meeting global nutrition, health, and survival goals, as well as economic growth and environmental sustainability.

Breastfeeding should be started within the first hour after delivery, continued exclusively for the first 6 months of life, and continued with safe and appropriate complementary foods for another 2 years or more, according to WHO and UNICEF.

Immediate and uninterrupted skin-to-skin contact and breastfeeding initiation within the first hour after birth are critical for breastfeeding establishment, as well as newborn and child survival and development.

When compared to neonates who were put to the breast within the first hour after birth, the risk of dying in the first 28 days of life is 33% greater for those who started breastfeeding 2-23 hours after delivery and more than twice as high for those who started 1 day or longer after birth. Early beginning provides protection till the age of 6 months.

Breastfeeding exclusively for six months offers the nurturing, nourishment, and energy required for physical and neurological growth and development.

Breastfeeding continues to deliver energy and high-quality nutrients after 6 months, which, when combined with safe and appropriate supplemental feeding, can prevent hunger, undernutrition, and obesity. Breastfeeding provides infants with food security.

Breastfeeding practices that are inadequate have a major negative impact on the health, development, and survival of newborns, children, and mothers.

"Breastfeeding is an essential component of realizing every child's right to the best possible health, while also respecting every mother's right to make an informed decision about how to feed her baby, based on complete, evidence-based information that is free of commercial interests, and the necessary support to enable her to carry out her decision."

BENEFITS OF BREASTFEEDING TO NURSING MOTHERS

Breastfeeding appears to profit both mothers and children's health, according to exploration.

A mother grows physically and emotionally as a result of her relationship with her baby. Just as a woman's breast milk is designed to nurture a child's body, the product and delivery of this milk benefits her own health.

Breast milk is always fresh, absolutely clean, and at the right temperature, and it's the healthiest option at the smallest possible cost.

•Breastfeeding is simple, indeed it does need some original literacy and adaptation for both mother and child.

•Breastfeeding is a low- cost system of feeding an invigorated, delivering the finest nutrition for the child at a low nutrient cost to the mother .

•Breastfeeding is doable during gestation, but milk product will probably drop at some point.

•Although breastfeeding is a system of birth control, it can delay the return of fertility through lactational amenorrhea. cling

•By breastfeeding, helpful hormones are produced into the mother 's body, which helps ameliorate the motherly relationship.

•A woman's capacity to produce all of the nutrients her child need can give her confidence. Suckling hormones contribute to the strengthening of the motherly attachment.

•According to experimenters, the link between a nursing mother and her child is lesser than any other mortal hassle.

Holding the child to her breast is a more profound cerebral experience for mothers than carrying the fetus within her uterus. Breastfeeding relations give the foundation of the mother - child relationship. The mother 's emotional health may be bettered by the relationship she creates with her child during breastfeeding, performing in lower anxiety and a stronger sense of connection with her baby.

This feeling establishes the health and cerebral foundation for the coming times. Expression of breast milk still, another guardian may be suitable to feed the baby expressed breast milk, If the mother isn't available. Working women can give their baby breast milk for as long as they want, thanks to the different breast pumps for easy extraction of milk.

To be successful, the mother must produce and save enough milk to feed the child during her absence, and the feeding guardian must be familiar with handling breast milk.

Breastfeeding causes the release of oxytocin and prolactin, which relax the mother and make her feel more caring towards her child. suckling soon after delivery raises the mothers ' oxytocin saw situations, causing her uterus to contract and recover to normal size briskly and minimizing bleeding.

Pitocin is a synthetic hormone that's structurally analogous to oxytocin and is used to constrict the uterus during and after labor.

Breastfeeding mothers are more likely to recapture their pre-pregnancy weight than formula feeding mothers.

Breastfeeding lowers the chance of developing long- term obesity.

Breastfeeding appears to minimize rotundity and hypertension threat. Because the fat gained during gestation is utilized to produce milk, nursing for at least 6 months can help mothers exfoliate weight.

Still, weight loss in nursing women is largely changeable; diet monitoring and adding the quantum/ intensity of exercise are more dependable strategies of reducing weight. Lactation causes mothers to burn a lot of calories while their bodies produce milk. In fact, some of the weight gained during gestation is used to fuel lactation. "

THE EFFECTS OF BREASTFEEDING IN MOTHERS

On return to gestation weight was negligible, and the effect of suckling on postpartum weight loss was unclear," according to a 2007 AHRQ analysis. Helps Birth Space Exclusive nursing reduces total implicit fertility in developing nations as much as all other ultramodern contraception styles combined.

Breastfeeding allows the mother to recover between gravities by distance from them. Postpartum Fertility on its

Own In the absence of period, exclusive nursing for the first 6 months postpartum is 98 percent effective in precluding gestation(similar to oral contraceptives), It's fully natural and free. The Lactation Amenorrhea Method(LAM) is used in this situation.   The following are mothers benefits of Breastfeeding:

•Emotional Well- Being: Because of the closeness of this relationship with the baby and the satisfaction of helping to nurture their kiddies, numerous mothers gain emotional benefits from nursing. At one month postpartum, women who breastfed their babies had lower anxiety and advanced mutuality scores than women who bottle fed their babies.

• According to several studies, mothers who breastfeed their babies have lower cases of postpartum depression.

• Breastfeeding soothes a toddler who's sick, agitated, bad, or injured. During those times, extended nursing can make mothering a toddler simpler(LLL).

• By making the mother sit or lie down with the child every many hours to feed, it allows the mother to gain important-demanded rest.

• Breastfeeding mothers report cerebral benefits similar to better tone- confidence and a better sense of connection with their babies.

•Breastfeeding is also encouraged in numerous countries and societies, which might help a new mother .

Eventually, breastfeeding provides babies with a healthy launch in life. Breastfeeding is a natural and healthy exertion for both mother and baby, numerous mothers are making the decision since it has significant health benefits for both the child and the mother , as well as emotional, profitable, and environmental benefits.

Lactation necessitates significant modifications in maternal metabolism in many species, notably high-producing dairy cattle and laboratory mice, in order to devote a major portion of metabolic output to milk synthesis.

These adaptations are especially impressive in certain animals, such as whales, seals, and hibernating bears, who do not eat for the most of the lactation period. These animals experience accelerated hunger, shifting nutrient fluxes to milk production.

Summarily, Milk secretion is a powerful mechanism that happens in approximately 85% of postpartum women. According to anecdotal evidence, at least 97% of women may efficiently nurse their infants given assistance in nursing practices. Because, at least in Western societies, when children fail to grow on the breast, formula substitution is simple, the causes of breastfeeding failure are poorly researched.

CHAPTER 2

THE SCIENCE OF BREAST MILK

Breast milk is distinct due to heredity and dietary variances.

Feeding between conception and a child's second birthday establishes the foundation for overall health. Allergies, GI, respiratory, and ear infections are less prevalent in breastfed babies. They are also less likely to be overweight, lower chance of acquiring diabetes later in life, and to have a higher IQ.

Breastfeeding lowers the risk of childhood diseases such as diarrhea and pneumonia, as well as premature death, and it also lessens the nutritional impairment to cognitive development in early infancy.Researchers have lately linked newborn formula usage to a slew of serious, chronic diseases and ailments, including SIDS, obesity, leukemia, breast cancer, and asthma.

Recent research has also revealed that even modest volumes of breast milk contain a variety of microorganisms that are advantageous to newborn health.

Breastfeeding also lowers the incidence of postpartum hemorrhage and depression in women, who are also less likely to acquire diabetes or breast or ovarian cancer.

The World Health Organisation, the Centres for Disease Control and Prevention, and the American Academy of Paediatrics all recommend that newborns be nursed exclusively until six months of age, with nursing remaining an essential part of the infant's diet until he or she is at least two years old.

Meanwhile, the World Health Organisation has set a goal of increasing breastfeeding rates to 50% at 6 months of age by 2025. Only 25% of infants under the age of six months are breastfed as of 2020.

There is a wealth of studies that shows that one's breast milk is individualized and unique. Comparisons between mothers have repeatedly revealed differences in milk composition in terms of beneficial nutrients as well as hazardous pollutants. The composition of breast milk and the maternal diet are significantly connected. Breast milk nutritional levels have been demonstrated to be directly related to the infant's health and development.

Toxins transmitted through breast milk have the same effect on infant health.

Some Tests concentrate on key nutrients for which evidence suggests that maternal nutrition influences levels observed in breast milk.Purposefully some research opted in for nutrients testing for which there is no evidence of a link between food and amounts observed in breast milk, such as vitamin D, zinc, phosphorus, sodium, and selenium.

For those nutrients influenced by maternal nutrition, a change in the breastfeeding mother's diet, whether through food or supplementation, leads to a change in the composition of her breast milk.

Furthermore, studies have shown that diet changes might have an effect on the lipid and calorie content of breast milk in as little as four days.

UNDERSTANDING THE PHYSIOLOGY OF BREASTFEEDING

Lactation is the process of producing and secreting milk from the breasts, as well as the time when the mother is breastfeeding. Let's begin by reviewing breast physiology.

The breasts contain mammary glands, which are responsible for nursing in females. Mammary glands are made up of 12 to 20 lobes, each with numerous tiny lobules. These tiny lobules have grape-like clusters of alveoli and breast secretory epithelial cells, which create milk during lactation. The lactiferous ducts connect these alveoli, lobules, and lobes to form a separate lactiferous duct for each lobe, which opens separately to drain the milk produced during lactation. The lactiferous sinus is a dilated region deep to the areola where a little drop of milk accumulates or stays in a nursing mother and is expelled from the areola when the areola is pressed during feeding.

During pregnancy, the placenta secretes progesterone, estrogen, and human placental lactogen, whereas the pituitary gland secretes prolactin. These hormones now work together to encourage the development of breast tissue by increasing the number and size of alveoli and the formation of lactiferous ducts.

Prolactin also stimulates milk production, and during the later stages of pregnancy, the breasts produce colostrum, a thick yellowish fluid heavy in protein and immunological cells. However, high levels of progesterone and estrogen limit milk production during this stage in order to avoid losing milk before the baby is born.

During pregnancy, the body begins to release many hormones that aid in the growth and development of the baby as well as the preparation of the breasts for milk production. Some of the physiological processes that occur during pregnancy are as follows.

•**Ductal Growth:** The mammary gland's ducts begin to divide and generate new branches. This is caused by estrogen hormone stimulation. Oestrogen also contributes to fat deposition.

•**Lobulo-alveolar Development:** As a result of duct branching, the alveolus at the duct terminal begins to develop. Progesterone hormone stimulation causes this.

•**Prolactin:** The hormone prolactin is produced in the body beginning with fertilization. This hormone regulates milk secretion but does not produce milk until the baby is delivered. This inhibition is caused by the hormones estrogen and progesterone.

The anterior pituitary gland is in charge of producing prolactin hormone. HPL, progesterone, and prolactin all work together to prepare alveolar cells for milk production.

The estrogen and progesterone hormone levels begin to diminish after the baby is born. In addition to the placenta, the body excretes estrogen and progesterone hormones. Lactogenesis, or milk secretion, is induced by the prolactin hormone.

Milk Composition.

Milk is a multi-phase fluid that can be divided by physical forces.

Membrane-bound globules (milk-fat globules) carrying milk lipids rise to the surface after many hours of sitting or with short-term, low-speed centrifugation, generating the cream layer that covers the skim milk. Fat encompasses milk components such as cholesterol, phospholipids, and steroid hormones and accounts for approximately 4% of milk volume in human and bovine milk23.

Regulation Of Milk Synthesis, Secretion, And Ejection.

Until milk withdrawal from the breast begins, milk is constantly synthesized and stored in the alveolar lumen. Two layers of regulation are required: (1) rate of synthesis and secretion regulation and (2) milk ejection regulation. Although these processes are ultimately dependent on baby sucking or other nipple stimulation, the mechanisms involved are diverse, both central and local. The CNS regulates milk secretion via prolactin, but its influence is

Oxytocin, Milk Ejection, And Suckling.

In conjunction with infant sucking, milk is withdrawn from the breast by contraction of myoepithelial cells, the processes of which form a basketlike network encircling the alveoli where milk is stored.

When newborns suckle, afferent impulses from sensory stimulation of nerve terminals in the areolus go to the CNS, where they stimulate the production of oxytocin from the posterior pituitary. In women, oxytocin release is typically associated with cues such as sight or sound.

HORMONES, STRESS, AND BREASTFEEDING.

Breastfeeding is usually recognised as one of the most difficult and spectacular acts accomplished by the human body. You've not only birthed a baby, but your body is now in charge of creating sustenance for it as well.

Breastfeeding and hormones have an essential and intricate relationship: your breast milk includes very specific hormones that flow into you. Your nursing experience also has an impact on your hormones in other ways, and these bodily functions might disrupt your postpartum biology.

Hormones Contained In Breast Milk

Breast milk contains a variety of hormones, both those that flow into your body and those that the infant consumes.

•**Prolactin**: Prolactin is the hormone that causes breast milk to be produced. It is present in extraordinarily high concentrations in colostrum, the initial type of breast milk produced after birth.

After a few days of breastfeeding, prolactin levels in breast milk drop considerably, and they are about equal to those seen in blood.

Thyroxine (T4): Thyroxine (T4) is a thyroid hormone generated by the thyroid gland (which is in charge of several vital biological activities, including metabolism and energy production). T4 levels in breastmilk are relatively low in the early stages of breastfeeding, but gradually increase over the first few weeks.

T4 may help a newborn's intestines expand and mature, and breastfed babies have substantially higher levels of thyroxine in their bodies than formula-fed infants do throughout the first few months of life.

•**Epidermal Growth Factor (EGF):** EGF stimulates cell growth and is especially crucial for the development of the infant digestive system. It is found in blood, saliva, breast milk, and amniotic fluid. Colostrum also includes large quantities of epidermal growth factor, but these levels drop rapidly after childbirth. Parents who have a premature infant will naturally have substantially higher amounts of EGF in their breast milk for the first month after delivery.

•**Cortisol:** also known as the "stress hormone," is one of the most well-known hormones. Cortisol levels in colostrum are high, but quickly decrease and remain low as breastfeeding continues. Unsurprisingly, studies have shown that cortisol levels in breast milk link to stress levels throughout the process - persons who have joyful, peaceful, positive breastfeeding experiences had lower amounts of cortisol in their breast milk.

According to research, the amount of cortisol in breast milk can also impact levels of a crucial antibody known as secretory immunoglobulin (sIgA), which helps protect a baby's immune system from illness and disease. Because high cortisol levels are related with lower sIgA levels, stress during nursing can interfere with the healthful, immune-protective qualities of breast milk.

It's no longer unusual that new mothers are encouraged to breastfeed their babies, citing the biological complexities of breast milk and the benefits it can provide for babies," the list continues. It's crucial to remember that moms should make breastfeeding decisions based on their own and their babies' health, and if breastfeeding becomes too stressful or physically challenging for them, forcing them to continue will not benefit either the baby or the mother. Medical advice is important to determine the best course of action to take.

Breastfeeding And Stress.

New mothers have a lot on their plates. It should come as no surprise that mothers sometimes feel their emotional and physical resources to cope are exhausted. This is known as stress, and it is an expected component of parenting

Some Stress Factors

You may feel overwhelmed as your hormones shift, as well as physical and psychological changes related to your new position as a mom.

However, additional factors such as your health status prior to and during pregnancy, the time of birth, your social or family environment, and your baby's health may all contribute to your stress levels. As if the list of potential causes wasn't extensive enough, nursing may also create stress.

What Effect Does Stress Have On Breastfeeding?

Breastfeeding is tough and time-consuming. Stress has an effect on both your milk supply and the contents of your milk. When you are stressed, your body responds by producing chemicals such as cortisol, adrenaline, and norepinephrine. While these may help you manage in the short term, they may have a negative long-term impact on your physical and mental health .

Maternal emotional anxiety suppresses the let-down reflex, which can result in milk flow disruption and lower milk volume. Mothers who are worried have more difficulty maintaining lactation.

If you are stressed or coping with a stressful circumstance and do not take the time to eat or drink enough water, or do not have the opportunity to breastfeed your baby as frequently as needed, it may reduce your milk production. The amount of milk your body produces is determined by how frequently your baby drinks. You will generate more if your baby drinks more.

What Effect Does Stress Have On Breast Milk Composition?

It is unclear how stress affects the nutrient composition of breast milk, however it may influence several immunological components in human milk and raise cortisol levels in breastmilk.

Don't worry, mother, here are some pointers to get you started:

•Stress reduction will benefit both you and your baba. Consider some of these relaxation suggestions.

•Stress Reduction Techniques

•Exercise releases endorphins, which may help you cope better with stress.

•Deep breathing techniques should be practiced.

•Call a friend or share your worries over a cup of tea.

•Set aside some time for yourself to do something you enjoy, such as reading a book.

•Play soothing music.

•Get as much sleep as you can.

•Request assistance. It is everyone's responsibility to raise children who will have a positive impact on the world.

•Make an effort to eat healthily, take care of yourself and your breastmilk. Mother balls are high in nutrients and require no preparation.

CHAPTER 3.

POSTPARTUM DEPRESSION AND BREASTFEEDING.

Much research has been conducted just to find out the missing link between Breastfeeding and postpartum depression. The two have a difficult relationship.While some research concluded that Breastfeeding protects against postpartum depression,some other research reveals that difficulties with Breastfeeding might lead a new mom to postpartum depression.

What Exactly Is Postpartum Depression?

Postpartum depression is a mental health issue that affects 13-19% of newly pregnant mothers. It is distinguished by a low mood as well as emotions of melancholy, hopelessness, and worthlessness.

It is important to distinguish postpartum depression from what is popularly referred to as "baby blues." Up to 80% of women experience baby blues. They relate to a brief time of mood changes following childbirth, such as irritation, worry, tearfulness, unhappiness with life, and sleep issues.

The baby blues normally go away within 10 days, but the emotional abnormalities linked with postpartum depression might continue much longer.

What Are The Ramifications Of Sad Mothers?

Postpartum depression can have a substantial impact on the mental health of mothers. Maternal depression increases the chance of developing various psychiatric illnesses such as anxiety disorder, panic disorder, and obsessive-compulsive disorder in women. Suicidal ideation (thoughts of killing oneself or the infant) is also common in mothers suffering from postpartum depression.

Another effect of the mother's bad mood is that it disrupts healthy mother-infant connection and bonding. As a result, postpartum depression can have an impact on an infant's social, emotional, physical, and cognitive development.

What Exactly Is The Connection Between Nursing And Postpartum Depression?

The connection between nursing and postpartum depression is not obvious. Initially, medical experts and researchers assumed that postpartum depression caused early breastfeeding discontinuation and lower nursing duration.Recent study indicates that the association is indeed bidirectional.

While depressive symptoms in new moms might contribute to lower breastfeeding rates, not starting breastfeeding can raise the risk of postpartum depression.

Relationship Between Women's Mental Health And Breastfeeding.

Breastfeeding may be beneficial in preventing postnatal depression. According to research, women who have never developed a nursing attachment with their newborn are 2.4 times more likely to experience postpartum depression symptoms than women who give their infant breast milk.

Breastfeeding women report an improvement in their mood after feeding their child.

The Connection Between Breastfeeding And Postpartum Depression.

When compared to nursing mothers, bottle-feeding mothers are more likely to develop depression.

Mothers with entirely breastfed newborns had lower levels of depression symptoms than mothers with partially breastfed children or mothers with bottle-fed infants.

As a result, exclusive breastfeeding appears to benefit women's health by lowering perceived stress and despairs.

Practises of breastfeeding, length, and severity of depression symptoms

Postpartum depression symptoms may be linked to early unpleasant breastfeeding experiences. In other words, women who have breastfeeding issues, such as those who try but fail to breastfeed due to a lack of milk supply, are more likely to have postpartum depression.

Mothers suffering from postpartum depression are more likely to discontinue nursing prematurely. While adverse nursing experiences can influence the development of postnatal depression, they do not appear to be connected to the degree of depressive symptoms.

Breastfeeding failure does not appear to worsen postpartum depression.

The Link Between Breastfeeding And Prenatal Maternal Depression

Women who have prenatal depression (depressive symptoms prior to childbirth) have a lower intention to breastfeed and a lower initiation of nursing after the baby is born.

If a woman does not have depressed symptoms before giving birth, she has a lower risk of postpartum depression if she intends to breastfeed and begins nursing. Women who do not intend to breastfeed or do not begin nursing, on the other hand, are at a higher risk of postpartum depression.

So, What's The Bottom Line?

The research findings are mixed, but most studies show a link between nursing and postpartum depression.

Breastfeeding and postpartum depression interact due to a variety of complex psychological, social, and physiological factors.

Scientists believe there is a symbiotic association between postpartum depression and early discontinuation of nursing in women who have begun breastfeeding, but that successful breastfeeding lessens postpartum depression.

Furthermore, not only are depressive symptoms after delivery common, but prenatal depression around the time of delivery might contribute to decreased breastfeeding frequency and early discontinuation of breastfeeding practices.

Finally, studies demonstrate that increasing the frequency of breastfeeding can result in a considerable reduction in depression symptoms and an increase in good mood for many months or even years following childbirth.

Breastfeeding has numerous advantages for both infant and maternal health. However, it may not be appropriate for every mother, and it is OK to pursue alternative methods of feeding an infant. Healthcare providers should take the time to understand pregnant women's wishes and discuss the benefits and drawbacks of nursing with them in order to assist them understand their options and make the best decision.

Postpartum depression is a mental condition that can occur whether or not a woman chooses to breastfeed. There are numerous drugs and therapies available to assist women suffering from depression symptoms. Antidepressant medicine, for example, may help a depressed mother to continue breastfeeding.

Discuss with your professional health provider if depression is blocking your ability to Breastfeed your child.

THE ROLE OF OXYTOCIN IN MOTHER AND CHILD BONDING .

Parent-infant bonding is commonly regarded as the basis for the infant's social connection. The parent-infant link is regarded to be the evolutionary and neurological basis for our ability to develop social bonds that ensure physical and mental health and welfare throughout adulthood.

Bio-behavioural provisions help to organize the newborn's physiological systems, stress reaction, and social orientation as parents engage with their infant. As researchers become more interested in biomarkers that promote bonding, caregiving, and synchrony, oxytocin (OT) has emerged as a major focus, as it has been discovered to play an important role in the developing nervous system and in the expression of sociality, both of which are critical to the development of relationships.

Oxytocin is a nine-amino-acid neuropeptide that is synthesized in the hypothalamus, travels to and is stored in the posterior pituitary gland, and has been found to increase activation in brain areas associated with bonding and empathy, as well as functional connections across those areas.

The limbic and neocortical systems - those structures associated with emotion - rely on early caregiving experiences to organize oxytocin availability. Neurobiologically, oxytocin drives the early child to preferentially select species-specific social stimuli to create dyadic attachments and is thought to be important in experience-dependent plasticity to feed forward auto-regulated functioning during key developmental phases.

Oxytocin aids in the regulation of the autonomic nerve system, which has implications for the sensory, visceral, metabolic, and smooth motor systems. Through the hypothalamus pituitary adrenal (HPA) axis, oxytocin improves social sensitivity and modifies responsiveness to stressors.

The HPA axis is an eloquent and dynamic intertwining of the neurological and endocrine systems. HPA function or dysfunction is mostly determined by genetics, early-life settings, and current life stress. Cortisol can be released for several hours in reaction to stress. Organisms become used to continuous HPA axis activity after repeated exposure to stimuli.

Oxytocin is found in a subgroup of neurons that respond to key adaptive or stress hormones, which regulate the HPA axis and have been linked to some of the negative effects of chronic stress. Oxytocin may be co-released as an adaptive response to a variety of positive and negative stressors. Oxytocin can promote emotional states that promote optimum growth and social skills.

Oxytocin may protect and mend tissues, as well as having antioxidant and anti-inflammatory characteristics that help buffer the effects of stress and adversity.

Numerous animal and human research have been conducted to examine parent-infant connection. Prairie voles have been used to study how early infant-parent interactions influence later social bonding abilities. Voles exposed to bi-parental licking and grooming outperformed those raised solely by the mother in terms of social bonding.

Another rodent study discovered that oxytocin influenced behavior, as maternal rats with high levels of Licking, Grooming, and Arch-Backed Nursing behaviors (LG-ABN) had higher oxytocin receptor densities in brain structures associated with oxytocin release than maternal rats with low LG-ABN levels. It appears that oxytocin is important in forming a strong parent-infant attachment as a result of the calming and reassuring interactions infants get during their early life care.

This has contributed to the understanding that parent-infant contact is essential for forming affiliative relationships. These connections are generated as a result of synchronous (or reciprocal) social encounters. Synchronous interactions occur when a parent or newborn responds to one another; the actions and responses are not preset and function as self-organizing processes based on the social inputs discovered in the encounter.Parental touch is important not just for social interaction but also for an infant's growth. Infant neurodevelopmental outcomes are influenced by the presence or absence of various early life experiences.

The social context of an infant's brain development is crucial. Neurobiological processes, such as genetic and/or epigenetic control, alter the infant's brain structure and functioning, which is dependent on experiences in order to improve the infant's emotional and self-regulation. The goal of this passage is to summarize the results of oxytocin research on the relationship between oxytocin levels and interactions between newborns and their parents.

In Conclusion, according to the review, oxytocin is vital in the establishment of bonding between infants and parents through early contact and interaction. Neurobiological, genetic, and social variables all contribute to the intricacies of oxytocinergic pathways.

CHAPTER 4

COMMON BREASTFEEDING ISSUES AND POSSIBLE SOLUTIONS

Breastfeeding can be difficult, especially in the early stages.But keep in mind that you are not alone. Lactation consultants can assist you in determining how to make nursing work for you and your baby. Some women experience a variety of issues during nursing, while others do not.

Furthermore, many women may experience issues with their first child that they may not experience with their second or third child. Some of these issues are listed below:

•Sore Nipples :

Many mothers report that their nipples are sore when they first begin breastfeeding. Breastfeeding should feel natural once you and your baby have discovered a good latch and a few positions that work for you.

Solution:

•Your kid should not suckle just from the nipple. Most of the areola (the darker coloured area around the nipple) and the nipple should be nursing.

•A good latch is essential; gradually break your baby's suction on your breast by inserting a clean finger into the corner of his or her mouth. Then, try once more to get your baby to latch on. (When your baby's nipple comes out of his or her mouth, it should be round and long, or the same shape as it was before the feeding.)

•If you are putting off feedings because breastfeeding is uncomfortable, seek the advice of a lactation expert. Delaying feedings might aggravate your pain and reduce your milk supply.

•Change positions every time you breastfeed.
Keep your broken nipples wet so you can keep breastfeeding. Try any of the following suggestions:

•After breastfeeding, gently rub a few droplets of milk on your nipples with clean fingertips. Human milk has natural healing qualities and soothing oils.

•Use pure lanolin cream or ointment designed specifically for breastfeeding.

•Allow your nipples to dry naturally after feeding, or use a soft cotton shirt.

•Before using creams, hydrogel pads (a moist covering for the nipple to assist relieve pain), or a nipple shield (a plastic device that shields the nipple during breastfeeding), ask your doctor or lactation consultant. These goods should not be used in certain situations. Your doctor or lactation consultant will assist you in making the best decision for you.

•Wear no bras or anything that is excessively tight and puts pressure on your nipples.

•Change nursing pads (washable or disposable pads that can be placed in your bra to absorb leaks) frequently to avoid moisture buildup that can lead to cracked nipples.

•On your nipples, avoid using harsh soaps or ointments containing astringents (such as toner). To keep your nipples and breasts clean, simply wash them with clean water.

•If your nipples are extremely painful, consult your doctor about non-aspirin pain treatments.

•Insufficient Milk Supply:

Most women produce an abundance of milk for their infants. However, many mothers are concerned about having enough milk. According to this video, the best approach to ensure your kid gets enough milk is to monitor his or her weight and progress. If you are concerned, notify your baby's doctor.

There may be occasions when you believe your supply is depleted, yet it is actually adequate:

Your breasts may no longer feel full when your baby is 6 weeks to 2 months old. This is typical. Your infant may only nurse for five minutes at a time at the same time. This could indicate that you and your baby are just becoming used to — and adept at — breastfeeding.

Growth spurts may cause your infant to nurse longer and more frequently. These growth spurts typically occur at 2 to 3 weeks, 6 weeks, and 3 months of age.

Growth spurts can occur at any time. Don't be concerned that your supply is insufficient to please your infant. Take your cues from your baby. Nursing more frequently will help you improve your milk supply. You'll probably be back to your old routine once your supply increases.

Solution:

•Properly check and Position your baby

•Breastfeed frequently and allow your baby to decide when to stop.

•At each feeding, provide both breasts. Allow your baby to remain at the first breast for as long as he or she is sucking and swallowing. When the baby slows or quits, offer the second breast.

•Avoid supplementing your baby's breastmilk with formula or cereal, especially during the first 6 months of life. Your baby's interest in your breastmilk may wane, and your milk production may drop. If you need to add more milk to your baby's feedings, use a spoon, cup, or dropper loaded with pumped breastmilk.

•If the following steps do not help, consult your doctor about health conditions such as hormone imbalances or primary breast insufficiency.

•**Milk Oversupply:**

Breastfeeding with an overfull breast can be stressful and difficult for both you and your baby.

Solution:

Breastfeed on one side at a time. Continue to offer that same breast for at least two hours before the next complete feeding, progressively extending the time per feeding.

•Hand express for a few moments to ease some of the pressure on the other breast if it seems unbearably full before you are ready to breastfeed on it. To relieve pain and swelling, apply a cool compress or washcloth.

•To avoid forceful sucking, feed your infant before he or she becomes extremely hungry.

•If your infant is gassy, burp him or her frequently to make more place in the gut for milk.

•Strong Let-down Reflex:

Some women have a powerful milk ejection reflex, often known as a let-down. This can occur in conjunction with an excess of milk.

Solution:

•Hold your nipple with the side of your hand or between your first and middle fingers. To lessen the force of milk ejection, lightly press on the milk ducts.

•If your infant chokes or sputters during breastfeeding, unlatch him or her and spritz any excess milk into a towel or cloth.

•Allow your infant to latch and unlatch from the breast at his or her leisure.

•Consider positions that lessen the force of gravity, which may heighten milk spray. The side-lying position and the football hold are examples of these positions.

•Engorgement :

When your breasts start producing milk, they will get larger, heavier, and more delicate. This fullness can sometimes progress to engorgement, which causes your breasts to feel quite firm and painful.

Building up of milk causes Engorgement and can also result in:

•Breast enlargement
•Breast sensitivity
•Warmth
•Redness
•Throbbing
•The nipple is flattening.
•Fever of low severity

Engorgement can result in clogged ducts or a breast infection, therefore it is critical to try to avoid it before it occurs.

Solution:

•After giving birth, breastfeed frequently. Allow your baby to feed for as long as he or she wants as long as he or she is latched on and sucking well.

•Consult a lactation expert to improve your baby's latch so that he or she can extract more milk from your breast.

•Breastfeed on the engorged side frequently to eliminate the milk, keep the milk circulating freely, and keep your breast from becoming overly full.

•Pacifiers or bottles should not be used to supplement feedings at first. Wait until your infant is 3 or 4 weeks old before introducing pacifiers.

•Before nursing, hand express or pump a little milk to soften the breast, areola, and nipple.

•Massage your breasts to relieve pain, apply cold compresses to your breasts in between feedings.

•If you're going back to work, attempt to pump your milk on the same timetable as your baby. Pump at least every four hours, if not more frequently.

•Get adequate rest, diet, and hydration.

•Wear a supportive, well-fitting bra that is not too tight.

Reverse pressure softening might help your infant latch by softening the areola near the base of the nipple. Try one of the holds shown in the diagrams below. Slowly count to 50 while pressing inward towards the chest wall. Apply consistent, forceful pressure while remaining soft enough to avoid pain. For a few days, you may need to do this every time you breastfeed.

One-handed "flower hold" works best with short fingernails. Curve your fingertips inward and place them where the baby's tongue will be.

Two-handed, one-step technique.It works best with short fingernails. Place your fingertips on each side of the nipple, curving them in towards your body.

Two-handed, one-step technique.You can ask someone to assist you by placing their fingers or thumbs on top of yours.

Two-handed, two-step technique.Place your first knuckles on either side of the nipple and move them 1/4 turn with two or three fingers on each side. Repeat the process above and below the nipple.

Two-handed, two-step technique.Place your thumbnails evenly on either side of the nipple with straight thumbs. Repeat 1/4 turn above and below the nipple.

The soft-ring technique.Place the areola on top of the bottom portion of an artificial nipple. Use your fingers to press it.

•Clogged Ducts:

Breastfeeding women frequently experience clogged ducts. A clogged milk duct feels like a painful lump in the breast. If you have a fever or other symptoms, you are most likely suffering from a breast infection rather than clogged ducts.

When a milk duct does not drain properly, it becomes clogged. Pressure then builds up behind the plug, inflaming the surrounding tissue. A blocked duct occurs in only one breast at a time.

Solution:

•Breastfeed every two hours on the side with a blocked duct. This will assist in loosening the blockage and keeping your milk flowing freely.

•Aim the chin of your infant at the plug. This will direct his or her suck to the damaged duct.

•Massage the affected area, beginning behind the aching point. Massage the nipple with your fingers in a circular motion. Apply a warm compress to the hurting spot.

Rely on others to assist you in getting more sleep, or rest with your feet up to aid in healing. A clogged duct is frequently an indication that you are doing too much.

•Wear a supportive, well-fitting bra that is not too tight, as a tight bra can choke milk ducts. Consider wearing a bra with no underwire.
Consult a lactation counselor if you have clogged ducts that keep returning.

•**Breast Infection (Mastitis)** :

Mastitis (mast-EYE-tiss) is a lump or pain in the breast. It can induce the following symptoms:

•Fever and/or flu-like symptoms, such as feeling exhausted or achy
•Nausea
•Vomiting
•Yellowish discharge from the breast resembling colostrum
•Breasts that are pink or red and feel warm or hot to the touch

A breast infection might occur while other family members are sick with a cold or the flu. It normally affects only one breast. It can be difficult to distinguish between a breast infection and a clogged duct because both have similar symptoms and can resolve within 24 to 48 hours. Some breast infections that do not resolve on their own require the use of a doctor's prescription medication. (For additional information about drugs and breastfeeding, see the Breastfeeding fact sheet.)

Solution:

•Every two hours or more, breastfeed on the affected side. This keeps the milk moving smoothly and prevents your breast from growing overly full.

•Massage the affected area, beginning behind the aching point. Massage the nipple with your fingers in a circular motion.
With a warm, damp cloth, apply heat to the hurting area.

•Rely on others to assist you in getting more sleep, or rest with your feet up to aid in healing. A breast infection is frequently a symptom that you are doing too much and growing exhausted.

•Wear a supportive, well-fitting bra that is not too tight, as a tight bra can choke milk ducts.

If you do not feel better after 24 hours of attempting these methods, if you have a fever, or if your symptoms worsen, consult your doctor. You could require medication. Seek immediate medical attention if :

•You appear to have a breast infection in both breasts.
•Your breast milk contains pus or blood.
•You have crimson stripes on your breast near the affected area.
•Your symptoms appeared abruptly and badly.

•Fungal Infections:

Yeast infections or thrush, popularly caused by a fungal infection can pop out on the nipple or breast.This infection feeds on milk and is caused by an overgrowth of the Candida bacterium.

Candida lives in our bodies and is kept healthy and at the proper levels by our bodies' natural flora. Candida can overgrow when the natural balance of bacteria is disturbed, resulting in infection.

Sore nipples that continue more than a few days, even after your baby has a good latch, are a significant symptom of a fungal infection. Or, after several weeks of pain-free breastfeeding, you may get sensitive nipples. Pink, flaky, glossy, itchy, or cracked nipples, as well as deep pink and blistered nipples, are further symptoms. You may also experience aching breasts or shooting pains deep within the breasts during or after feedings.

•The following are some of the causes of fungal infection:
•Thrush in your baby's mouth, which you can catch
•Bruised or cracked nipples
Antibiotics or steroids (which are frequently given to moms during labor)
•A chronic ailment, such as HIV, diabetes, or anemia

Solution:

A drug that you spread on your breasts several times a day for about a week is used to treat fungal infections. It may take several weeks for the illness to heal up, thus it is critical to follow these precautions to avoid spreading it:

•Replace disposable nursing pads on a regular basis.

•Any towels or clothing that has come into touch with the yeast should be washed in very hot water (over 122°F).

•Every day, wear a clean bra.

•Wash your hands frequently.

•If your baby sucks on his or her fingers, wash his or her hands frequently.

•All pacifiers, bottle nipples, and toys that your infant puts in his or her mouth should be boiled every day. (To boil them, throw them in a pot of water and bring to a boil, then cook for about 10 minutes.)

•After one week of treatment, discard all pacifiers and nipples and replace them with new ones.

•Every day, boil all breast pump parts that come into contact with your milk.

•Check to see whether any other family members have thrush or other fungal illnesses. If they exhibit symptoms, do not let them care for you or your baby until they have been treated.

Inverted, Flat, Or Very Huge Nipple:

Some women have nipples that bend inside rather than outward, or they are flat and do not protrude. Nipples might also flatten for a brief period of time due to engorgement or swelling from nursing.

Breastfeeding can be made more difficult by inverted or flat nipples.

Breastfeeding requires your infant to latch onto both the nipple and the breast, therefore even inverted nipples can work. Flat and inverted nipples frequently protrude more when the baby sucks more.

Large nipples can make it difficult for the baby to get enough areola into his or her mouth to compress the milk ducts and obtain sufficient milk.

Solution:

•If you are concerned about your nipples, visit your doctor or a lactation specialist.

•Pull out your nipple with your fingers.

•You can also discuss utilizing a device that gently suctions or pulls out inverted or temporarily flattened nipples with your doctor or nurse.

As the baby grows, the latch for newborns born to mothers with particularly large nipples will improve. It may take several weeks for the baby to latch properly. However, if you have a sufficient milk supply, your baby will get adequate milk even with a sloppy latch.

Nursing Strike:

A nursing "strike" occurs when your child has been successfully breastfeeding for months before abruptly refusing the breast.

A nursing strike could mean that your

child is trying to tell you that something is wrong. This may not always signify that the infant is ready to wean (totally cease breastfeeding).

Not all babies will react similarly to the many causes that can cause a breastfeeding strike. Some babies will keep breastfeeding normally. Other babies may simply get fussy at the breast. Other newborns will reject the breast totally.

Some of the primary causes of a nursing strike are as follows:

•Teething discomfort, a fungal infection like thrush, or a cold sore

•An ear infection that causes discomfort when sucking or pressure when sleeping on one side.

•Pain from a specific breastfeeding position, potentially due to a baby's physical injury, or soreness after a vaccination

•Being disturbed as a result of a long separation from one's mother or a big change in routine

•Being distracted when breastfeeding, for example, by observing what is going on around the baby

•Having a cold or congested nose that makes it difficult to nurse

•Receiving less milk from the mother after supplementing breast milk with bottles or excessively using a dummy

•Respond violently if the infant bites the mother while she is breastfeeding.

•Being annoyed by arguments or someone speaking loudly when breastfeeding.

You may be wanting to nurse as a result of stress, overstimulation, or being repeatedly put off. If your infant is on a nursing strike, it is natural to be frustrated and sad, especially if your baby is in pain. Continue to offer your breasts to your child while remaining gentle. You should also pump your breast milk throughout the strike to avoid becoming engorged.

Solution:

•Hand express or pump your milk as regularly as your baby used to breastfeed to minimize engorgement and plugged ducts.

•Use another feeding method, such as a cup, dropper, or spoon, to temporarily provide your breastmilk to your kid.

•Keep track of your baby's wet and dirty diapers to ensure that he or she gets enough milk.

•Continue to give your infant your breast. Take a break and try again later if your infant becomes frustrated. You can also try offering your breast to your infant if he or she is very sleepy or asleep.

•Experiment with nursing positions that include rubbing your bare skin against your baby's bare skin.

•Concentrate on your youngster and provide additional caressing and hugging.

•Breastfeed your infant while rocking him or her in a quiet, distraction-free atmosphere.

•Breastfeed your infant while rocking him

CHAPTER 5

COPING STRATEGIES FOR BREASTFEEDING MOTHERS.

Being a new parent can be challenging. The delight of cooing and cuddling is mixed in with the hard work of newborn care. It's normal to be frustrated and tired. Parenting becomes much more difficult if your infant is always crying or refuses to sleep.

During these early stages of parenthood, it's critical to take care of yourself by relying on family and friends as well as your pediatrician for assistance. Remember that you are not alone. Here is some information that may be useful.

Child Care:

Crying is typical for babies: babies cry an average of 2-3 hours each day throughout their first six weeks of life. Most babies begin crying excessively about two weeks of age and continue for about two months.

Soothing Suggestions: You may need to try a few different things to assist soothe your baby. To begin, try holding, feeding, swaddling, softly rocking, or singing to them. It can take some trial and error to figure out what works best for your infant. Some things may have to be attempted several times before they work.

If soothing does not work, place your baby on their back in a safe sleep environment (nothing in the bed but the baby on a hard sleep surface with a tight-fitting sheet, without any blankets, toys, pillows, or other material). While some newborns cry for an extended period of time, many parents are shocked by how quickly their kids cry themselves to sleep.

What if the baby refuses to sleep?

Until roughly six months of age, babies do not have regular sleep patterns. And some people only sleep for one or two hours at a time.

Here's what you should do if your infant is having problems falling asleep.

What about sibling conflict?

If you have other children, don't be surprised if they become hostile towards the newborn pending the time they would adjust. Make it plain to your children how to care for the new baby. Thank them for their assistance. Have lots of healthy distractions available for children, and try to keep your cool when things don't go as planned.

Personal Care:

Make an effort to rest yourself.It is critical that you take a rest. Sleep when the baby is asleep. Alternatively, ask your partner or another responsible adult to monitor your child while you take a break.

Stop putting yourself under pressure to be flawless.Remember that there is no "only" way to be a parent. Approaches and styles can differ. In addition, all parents require assistance and support.

Make contact with people.You may be sleepy most of the time, but talking with other adults is beneficial. Stay in touch with friends and family by using video chats or social media. This is especially essential during the COVID-19 pandemic, when social isolation can make new parents feel more alone.

Make use of your "helpers."Engage your baby's older siblings as much as possible by encouraging them to be your special assistants, so they may assist in age-appropriate ways.

If you require assistance, seek it.After having a baby, it is natural to have feelings of sadness or depression. If you had a history of depression before having your kid, you may be more prone to postpartum depression. Your pediatrician can assist you.

Look for a parent group.You might find it beneficial to discuss your concerns with other moms in your neighborhood or online. Sharing your experience with someone who is going through the same situation can be really beneficial.

Your pediatrician is here to assist you.Never be afraid to seek advice. Your pediatrician will comprehend your baby's needs as well as your situation.

Things To Abstain From As A Mother

•Alcohol is not the solution.It is not safe to care for a newborn while inebriated.

Drinking alcohol hinders your judgment and capacity to care for your infant securely. If you drink excessively, make arrangements for a sober adult to care for your kid at this time.

Lactation and alcohol.Alcohol enters your baby through your breast milk. The American Academy of Paediatrics advises breastfeeding mothers to abstain from alcohol.

The myth of the pump and dump.Expressing or pumping milk after consuming alcohol and then discarding it (sometimes known as "pumping and dumping") does not reduce the quantity of alcohol in your milk quickly. If alcohol is still present in your bloodstream, breast milk includes alcohol. As your blood alcohol level decreases, so does the amount of alcohol in your breast milk.

The importance of timing cannot be overstated.If you want to drink alcohol on occasion, it's preferable to do so after you nurse or pump milk, rather than before. It is safe to breastfeed or pump breast milk two hours after your last drink. Your body will have more time to remove itself of the alcohol, and less of it will reach your infant.

Marijuana And Breastfeeding : These are not compatible.There is no amount of marijuana that is safe to use during pregnancy or breastfeeding. Marijuana toxins can transfer via your breastmilk to your kid, impairing your capacity to care for him or her.

In conclusion,alcohol and pregnancy.If you are considering having another child, keep in mind that no amount of alcohol during pregnancy is risk-free. No type of alcohol is risk-free during pregnancy. And there is no moment when alcohol drinking is risk-free during pregnancy.

NUTRITION AND SELF-CARE FOR NURSING MOTHERS.

Breastfeeding women frequently overlook the importance of caring for themselves as well as their children. There's so much to think about with remembering when the baby last fed, ensuring the baby's placement and latch are correct, and tracking dirty diapers that it's easy to neglect your own well-being.

However, it is critical to consider both your own and your child's requirements. Here are some self-care tips for breastfeeding parents, covering nutrition, weight loss, exercise, hygiene, and emotional wellness.

•**Nutrition:** There are numerous myths and old wives' tales regarding what breastfeeding women should and should not consume, but you can pretty much disregard them all. It's fine to eat broccoli, garlic, onions, spicy foods, citrus, and even chocolate in moderation. What matters most is that you acquire the nutrition your body requires when breastfeeding.

•Keep taking your prenatal vitamins.
•Stay hydrated by drinking plenty of water.
•Consume a nutritious, well-balanced diet.
•Consume 500 additional calories per day.1

If your food is nutritionally deficient, you will sacrifice nutrients from your own body. Your body will take what it needs to generate nutritious breast milk for your baby first, leaving you with whatever is left over, leaving you feeling depleted and fatigued.

You may keep your body healthy and strong while producing breast milk by consuming a variety of foods and choosing nutritious food and snack choices. You should also eat items that you enjoy. For less healthful foods, simply consume them in moderation as part of a well-balanced diet.Breastfeeding Nutritional Needs

Loss of Pounds: Breastfeeding may aid in weight loss, but postpartum weight loss is dependent on your body and food. Here are some suggestions for staying healthy during nursing.

You should lose weight gradually while breastfeeding if you eat a nutritious, well-balanced diet.In general, losing weight gradually is the healthiest option. The safe limit is usually thought to be no more than one pound each week. If you believe you need to drop additional weight, consult your doctor and wait until your child is at least two months old.

By two months, your milk supply has had time to establish itself, and more considerable weight loss will not be as shocking to your body.

Remember that what you eat can have an impact on your capacity to lose weight. Your body requires more calories while breastfeeding, but if you consistently consume more calories than your body requires, you will gain weight.

Focus on nourishing your body with nutritious foods and keeping healthy, enjoyable snacks within arm's reach of where you nurse the most. Adding exercise to a balanced diet can also aid in weight loss. Consult your doctor about beginning light to moderate activity.

While decreasing the weight gained during pregnancy is a reasonable aim for many new moms, it's also critical to avoid dropping too much weight too rapidly. Rapid weight loss can result in a decrease in milk production.Avoid calorie-restricted diets and any weight loss products, pills, or supplements for your own and your baby's sake.

If you decide to start a weight loss programme, be sure you're eating enough calories each day and that your doctor is keeping track of your progress.

Every woman is unique. While it is natural to desire to reduce the weight you gained during pregnancy after giving birth, it is critical to be patient and give yourself time.Safe Weight Loss While Breastfeeding

Physical Activity: It may seem like it will be years before you can return to the gym after having a child. However, exercise is essential for your health as a breastfeeding mother. Of course, with tiredness levels at an all-time high, a 5K run is certainly out of the question. You can, however, make it a daily goal to go for a great, quick walk.

Instead of pushing yourself to accomplish grandiose fitness goals, concentrate on finding doable, sustainable exercise that you love and makes you feel good. Here are some suggestions to consider when exercising while breastfeeding:

Before you begin exercising, breastfeed (or pump) your baby: If your breasts aren't excessively full with breast milk, your workout will be more comfortable.

Take in every second of your "you time" and workout. Serotonin, a mood-boosting hormone, will be released into your body as you do so.So, even if this is your only outing for the day, you may still feel like a million bucks.

Maintain adequate hydration, especially in hot weather: Drink at least 64 ounces of water per day. Drink much more if you're perspiring profusely during your workout.

Take a shower or wash your breasts after you exercise and before you breastfeed to remove sweat from your breasts and nipples. Sweat has a salty taste that some newborns dislike.

Wear The Proper Bra: You need support, but you don't want it to be excessively tight or have an underwire. Anything that puts too much strain on your breast tissue can trigger clogged milk ducts or mastitis.Your Exercise and Breastfeeding Handbook

Taking Care of Your Breasts: There isn't much you can do to care for your breasts when breastfeeding, but there are a few things you can do to keep comfortable and avoid breast problems.

While nursing, it's critical to practice good hygiene, which includes having a daily shower or bath and wiping your breasts. Nursing mothers have been taught for years not to wash their breasts with soap because it will dry out the nipple area. However, if you use a gentle, moisturizing soap and completely rinse it off, this should not be an issue.

Natural oils secreted by the Montgomery glands—the small bumps visible on your areola—cleanse and moisturize the nipples when breastfeeding. They also aid in the prevention of bacterial reproduction. You don't want to interfere with these glands' function, so only lightly wash the breasts.

Because breast milk has anti-infective characteristics, it's also useful to rub some of your expressed breast milk into your nipples and let it air dry.

Wear a fresh, clean nursing bra every day, and change it if it becomes filthy or damp during the day. Also, if you use breast pads to absorb leaky breast milk, make sure to change them frequently.

Skin breakdown might occur if you have a wet bra or damp breast pads on your breasts. Furthermore, the warm, moist, sugary atmosphere is ideal for the growth of bacteria or yeast.If you experience unpleasant breast concerns, such as sore nipples or clogged milk ducts, address them as soon as possible to avoid them worsening or interfering with nursing.

Emotional and Mental Well-Being: In a matter of minutes, new mothers can shift from happy to unhappy and back again. There might be a lot of unexpected emotions, from changing hormones to weariness to cradling your new bundle of joy. It's quite normal to have a variety of emotions. Here are some suggestions for caring for your emotional and mental health while nursing.

Create A Support System: Breastfeeding can be extremely satisfying, but it can also be fraught with difficulties, anxiety, and failures. Consider the persons in your life to whom you can seek guidance and assistance. It might be your partner, mother, sibling, therapist, or a close friend.

Consider attending a local or online breastfeeding support group if you don't have a good support system. You never know when a breastfeeding problem will arise and you will require some assistance to get through it.6

Get Assistance: Breastfeeding is natural, but parents and babies may want assistance in getting started. You must both learn this critical new skill. It can be frustrating and bring up emotions of guilt or failure if you are having difficulty getting your baby to latch or if your infant is very sleepy.

Asking for assistance from the start will help get breastfeeding off to a good start. And asking help when you need it will boost your confidence and set you and your baby on the road to breastfeeding success.Where Can I Get Breastfeeding Support?

Have Enough Rest: When you're a mum, you have a lot on your plate. Your everyday tasks might get daunting, and this is exacerbated when you are weary. It may be difficult to get adequate rest, but you can attempt. You'll feel healthier and more prepared to take on your obligations if you sleep when your baby sleeps and take every opportunity to put your feet up and close your eyes.

Discuss Your Emotions: You do not have to keep everything within. It is acceptable to feel the way you do, and talking about it can help you feel better. If you are unable to communicate with your partner, family, or friends, or if you do not feel comfortable communicating with them, you can consult a professional. Your doctor is an excellent resource and can put you in touch with the correct individual.Postpartum Depression vs. Postpartum Blues

Make Some Time for Yourself: Too frequently, mothers believe they must do everything. However, you are not required to do everything for everyone 24 hours a day, seven days a week. It is acceptable to set aside time for yourself. Allow your partner, a family member, or a friend to watch the baby while you go for a stroll, get a manicure, have lunch with a friend, or simply nap.

Taking time for yourself to do something you enjoy will help you to return to your invigorated responsibilities, which is beneficial to both you and your kid.

Get Ready for Weaning: You might not expect a wave of melancholy when it comes time to wean your kid. However, even if you were expecting or looking forward to the end of your breastfeeding relationship, it can be very tough.

By seeing and admitting the loss and transition, you may better prepare yourself to leave that period of your life with your child behind and look forward to the future adventures you will share as your child develops.

Postpartum Depression Symptoms: Breastfeeding mothers are likely to experience a wide range of typical emotions. Extreme grief, guilt, or anxiety, on the other hand, can be a sign of something more serious. Seek for medical attention if you are experiencing any of the listed below signs.

•Frequently crying
•Excessive concern or anxiety about parenting and your child
•Appetite loss
•Nursing the desire to hurt or harm yourself or your baby.
•Loss of interest in previously enjoyed activities
•Sleeping problems

In Conclusion, When you're a busy and fatigued new mum, it's easy to forget or put off caring for yourself. Setting aside some time each day to care for your physical and emotional wellbeing, on the other hand, is not selfish. It could be the most beneficial thing you can do for your family.

When you take care of your own needs by eating correctly, getting enough rest, taking a shower, and spending time with a friend, you will feel healthier and happier. And, while you're feeling good, you'll be more prepared and capable of caring for your infant and family.

SYNOPSIS AND CONCLUSION.

Investigating and dismantling the connection among nursing and new mothers' psychological well-being shows serious areas of strength for the connection between breastfeeding moms and their infants. The creation of oxytocin, otherwise called the "adoration chemical," while nursing diminishes pressure and upgrades the mother-kid bond.

In any case, nursing can cause entanglements that, whenever left untreated, could adversely affect a mother's emotional well-being.

Lactation management is a significant emotionally supportive network that gives training, guiding, and help in defeating concerns including hooking troubles and low milk creation. Lactation management assists mothers with encountering the profound benefits of nursing by defeating these deterrents, fabricating a unique bond with their infants.

Breastfeeding is a significant demonstration of adoration and bonding between a mother and her newborn child .

Nevertheless, it is essential to acknowledge that breastfeeding can significantly improve a mother's mental health. While oxytocin and profound bonds are valuable, nursing troubles can cause pressure and bitterness.

Therefore, lactation of the executives becomes basic. Lactation management urges mothers to defeat breastfeeding hindrances by providing guidance and backing, bringing about a cheerful encounter for both mother and youngster.

At last, the connection among breastfeeding and maternal psychological well-being is clear, and lactation the board is basic in supporting this tie. As we go further into this stand-out relationship, we find the science as well as the close to home side of nursing. With the right help, mothers can deal with and solve problems, enjoy nursing, and build a strong emotional bond with their children. The mother and the child will both benefit from this connection for a long time.